ABOUT US

Our vision at Links2Success is to duplicate our personal success for each of our clients. We do this by teaching the skills in demand by today's wellness minded patient. The business of dentistry is something most dentists are never taught to manage properly while attending dental school.

Our philosophy is to teach our clients how to become strong business leaders within the field of Oral Medicine. Training encompasses steps to increased profitability and delivery of a better patient experience, all while maximizing office efficiency.

ABOUT THE AUTHOR

Christine Taxin

Christine Taxin is the founder and president of Links2Success, a practice management consulting company to the dental and medical fields. Prior to starting her own consulting company Ms. Taxin served as an administrator of a critical care department at Mt. Sinai Hospital in New York City and managed an extensive multi-specialty dental practice in New York. With over 25 years' experience as a practice management professional she now provides private practice consulting services, delivers continuing education seminars for dental and medical professionals and serves as an adjunct professor at the New York University (NYU) Dental School and Resident Programs for Maimonides Hospital.

The information provided in this book is meant to inform and educate on the insurance rules and regulations for *The Dentist's Guide to Medical Billing – Oral & Maxillofacial Surgery*. It is correct and updated to the best of my ability, at the date of this publication. It is not meant to offer you legal advice or to be considered an all-inclusive source of insurance information or the rules of billing. Insurance companies, including Medicare, update and change rules and requirements without notification. If you join our school website you will have access to asking questions or to keep updated on changes as I learn them.

ORAL & MAXILLOFACIAL SURGERY

ORAL AND MAXILLOFACIAL SURGERY D7000 - D7999

Local anesthesia is usually considered to be part of Oral and Maxillofacial Surgical procedures.
For dental benefit reporting purposes a quadrant is defined as four or more contiguous teeth and/or teeth spaces distal to the midline.

General Guidelines

1. The fee for all oral and maxillofacial surgery includes local anesthesia, suturing if needed and postoperative care 30 days following surgery (e.g. dry socket, bleeding). Separate fees for these procedures when performed in conjunction with oral and maxillofacial surgery are disallowed when done by the same dentist/dental office and are denied and the approved amount is collectable from the patient when done by another dentist/dental office.

2. When a medical carrier statement is required, the procedure should be submitted to the patient's medical carrier first. When submitting to HDS, a copy of the explanation of payment or payment voucher from the medical carrier should be included with the claim, plus a narrative describing the procedure and reasons for performing the procedure, pathology report if appropriate, and any other information deemed pertinent. In the absence of such information, the procedure will not be benefited by HDS.

3. Medical carrier statement of payment is not required for HMO. Indicate the HMO name in a narrative.

4. Impaction codes are based on the anatomical position of the tooth, rather than the surgical procedure necessary for removal.

5. Exploratory surgery is denied.

6. Benefits are disallowed for incomplete or unsuccessful attempts at extractions.

7. Bone grafts in new extraction sites, with or without an implant, are denied as a specialized technique.

8. When submitting for surgical extraction(D7210) and the tooth is not cariously broken down, fractured, or otherwise compromised, the provider should submit a narrative that states the clinical reason(s) which prevented removal of the tooth via customary elevation and forceps.

9. When a "narrative" is required, the corresponding guidelines may state what is expected in the narrative. When "narrative" expectations are not specifically stated in the guidelines, the narrative must include:

    a. Diagnosis
        Example: Acute periapical abscess #30 with fluctuant swelling on buccal.

    b. Determination of Treatment (Brief description of the procedure performed)
        Example: I & D of Acute periapical abscess.

    c. Procedure or Treatment Performed (Steps of surgical procedure, to include location and instrument used)
        Example: Incision on buccal of #30 with #15 scalpel, drain placed and secured with one 3-0 black silk suture.

v.2019

ORAL & MAXILLOFACIAL SURGERY

Code & Nomenclature	Submission Requirements	Valid Tooth/ Quad/Arch/ Surface

Extractions (Includes local anesthesia, suturing, if needed, and routine postoperative care) D7111 - D7140

1. Under certain plans where Enhanced ACA Pediatric Benefits apply,or Patient has Medical Coverage the extraction, surgery must meet the medical necessity criteria in order to benefit. Medically Necessary Criteria include but are not limited to:
Non-restorable caries or fracture
Recurrent infection / Pericoronitis / cellulitis / abscess / osteomyelitis
Associated cysts/tumors
Resorption/damage to adjacent teeth
Damage/destruction of bone
Non-treatable pulpal / periapical pathology
Intenal/ external resorption of third molar
Ectopic position or eruption of third molar

D7111
extraction, coronal remnants – deciduous tooth

A - T

Removal of soft tissue-retained coronal remnants.

1. Includes soft tissue-retained coronal remnants.

2. D7111 is considered part of any other primary surgery in the same surgical area on the same date and the fee is disallowed if performed by the same dentist/dental office.

CROSS CODES
D7111
Extraction, coronal remnants - primary tooth

K05.20 Aggressive periodontitis, unspecified
K05.21 Aggressive periodontitis, localized
K09.0   Developmental odontogenic cysts

L03.90 Cellulitis, unspecified

R69   Illness, unspecified

S02.5XXA
Fracture of tooth (traumatic), initial encounter for closed fracture

41805 Removal of embedded foreign body from dentoalveolar structures; soft tissues
41899 Unlisted procedure, dentoalveolar structures

v.2019

ORAL & MAXILLOFACIAL SURGERY

Code & Nomenclature	Submission Requirements	Valid Tooth/ Quad/Arch/ Surface

Extractions (Includes local anesthesia, suturing, if needed, and routine postoperative care) D7111 - D7140

1. Under certain plans where Enhanced ACA Pediatric Benefits apply,or Patient has Medical Coverage the extraction, surgery must meet the medical necessity criteria in order to benefit. Medically Necessary Criteria include but are not limited to:
Non-restorable caries or fracture
Recurrent infection / Pericoronitis / cellulitis / abscess / osteomyelitis
Associated cysts/tumors
Resorption/damage to adjacent teeth
Damage/destruction of bone
Non-treatable pulpal / periapical pathology
Intenal/ external resorption of third molar
Ectopic position or eruption of third molar

D7140
extraction, erupted tooth or exposed root (elevation and/or forceps removal)

A - T,
1 - 32

Includes removal of tooth structure, minor smoothing of socket bone and closure, as necessary.

CROSS CODES
D7140
Extraction, erupted tooth or exposed root (elevation and/or forceps removal)

K05.20 Aggressive periodontitis, unspecified
K05.21 Aggressive periodontitis, localized
K09.0 Developmental odontogenic cysts

L03.90 Cellulitis, unspecified

R69 Illness, unspecified

S02.5XXA
Fracture of tooth (traumatic), initial encounter for closed fracture

41899
Unlisted procedure, dentoalveolar structures

ORAL & MAXILLOFACIAL SURGERY

Code & Nomenclature	Submission Requirements	Valid Tooth/ Quad/Arch/ Surface

Surgical Extractions (Includes local anesthesia, suturing, if needed, and routine postoperative care) D7210 - D7251

1. The fee for surgical extraction includes local anesthesia, suturing if needed, and postoperative care 30 days following surgery (e.g. dry socket, bleeding).

2. When the x-ray or other submitted documentation does not support the procedure code D7210, the procedure code will be processed as D7140.

3. Under certain plans where Enhanced ACA Pediatric Benefits apply, the extraction must meet the medical necessity criteria in order to benefit. Medically Necessary Criteria include but are not limited to:

- Non-restorable caries or fracture
- Recurrent infection / Pericoronitis / cellulitis / abscess / osteomyelitis
- Associated cysts/tumors
- Resorption/damage to adjacent teeth
- Damage/destruction of bone
- Non-treatable pulpal / periapical pathology
- Internal/ external resorption of third molar
- Ectopic position or eruption of third molar

Code & Nomenclature	Submission Requirements	Valid Tooth/ Quad/Arch/ Surface
D7210 Extraction, erupted tooth requiring removal of bone and/or sectioning of tooth, and including elevation of mucoperiosteal flap if indicated	X-ray	A - T, 1 - 32

Includes cutting of gingiva and bone, removal of tooth structure, minor smoothing of socket bone and closure.

1. When extracting a tooth that is not significantly broken down due to caries or fracture, the provider is requested to submit a narrative which details the reason(s) that prevented non-complicated removal via elevator/forceps.

2. Incisional biopsy of oral tissue – soft (D7286) and removal of benign odontogenic cyst or tumor up to 1.25cm (D7450) are subject to dental consultant review and may be disallowed in conjunction with this procedure.

CROSS CODES ON NEXT PAGE

v.2019

ORAL & MAXILLOFACIAL SURGERY

D7210

Extraction, erupted tooth requiring removal of bone and/or sectioning of tooth, and including elevation of mucoperiosteal flap if indicated

X-ray

A - T,
1 - 32

CROSS CODES
D7210
Extraction, erupted tooth requiring removal of bone and/or sectioning of tooth, and including elevation of mucoperiosteal flap if indicated = 41899 Unlisted procedure, dentoalveolar structures

K05.20 Aggressive periodontitis, unspecified
K05.21 Aggressive periodontitis, localized
K09.0   Developmental odontogenic cysts

L03.90 Cellulitis, unspecified

R69   Illness, unspecified

S02.5XXA
Fracture of tooth (traumatic), initial encounter for closed fracture

---

D7220

removal of impacted tooth – soft tissue

X-ray

A - T,
1 - 32

Occlusal surface of tooth covered by soft tissue; requires mucoperiosteal flap elevation.

CROSS CODES
D7220
Removal of impacted tooth - soft tissue

41899 Unlisted procedure, dentoalveolar structures

D7230

removal of impacted tooth – partially bony

X-ray

A - T,
1 - 32

Part of crown covered by bone; requires mucoperiosteal flap elevation and bone removal.

CROSS CODES
D7230
Removal of impacted tooth - soft tissue

41899 Unlisted procedure, dentoalveolar structures

ORAL & MAXILLOFACIAL SURGERY

Code & Nomenclature	Submission Requirements	Valid Tooth/ Quad/Arch/ Surface
D7240 removal of impacted tooth – completely bony	X-ray	A - T, 1 - 32

Most or all of crown covered by bone; requires mucoperiosteal flap elevation and bone removal.

1. For benefit purposes, completely bony is considered as 90% of the crown covered by bone.

CROSS CODES
D7240
Removal of impacted tooth - completely bony

41899 Unlisted procedure, dentoalveolar structures

Code & Nomenclature	Submission Requirements	Valid Tooth/ Quad/Arch/ Surface
D7241 removal of impacted tooth – completely bony, with unusual surgical complications	X-ray, Operative Report	A - T, 1 - 32

Most or all of crown covered by bone; unusually difficult or complicated due to factors such as nerve dissection required, separate closure of maxillary sinus required or aberrant tooth position.

1. Operative report **must** clearly indicate the specific complication/s incurred during the course of the surgical procedure.

2. When the operative report does not indicate the complication or difficulty incurred during the course of the surgical procedure, this service will be processed as D7240 or the appropriate procedure code.

CROSS CODES
D7241
Removal of impacted tooth - completely bony, with unusual surgical complications

K00.1 Supernumerary teeth
K05.20 Aggressive periodontitis, unspecified
K05.21 Aggressive periodontitis, localized
K09.0 Developmental odontogenic cysts

L03.90 Cellulitis, unspecified
R69 Illness, unspecified

41899 Unlisted procedure, dentoalveolar structures

v.2019

ORAL & MAXILLOFACIAL SURGERY

Code & Nomenclature	Submission Requirements	Valid Tooth/ Quad/Arch/ Surface
D7250 removal of residual tooth roots (cutting procedure)	X-ray	A - T, 1 - 32

Includes cutting of soft tissue and bone, removal of tooth structure, and closure.

1. This benefit applies only to retained sub-osseous root tips.

2. This benefit is disallowed if submitted in conjunction with a surgical extraction (in the same surgical area) by the same dentist/dental office.

3. When the submitted X-ray image or other documentation does not support the HDS clinical criteria for D7250, the procedure may be processed as noted below:

   - When the residual root is not fully encased in bone (sub-osseous), the procedure will be processed as either D7210 (surgical removal of erupted tooth) or D7140 (extraction, erupted tooth or exposed root) based on the clinical circumstances and submitted documentation.

CROSS CODES
D7250
Removal of residual tooth roots (cutting procedure)

K00.1 Supernumerary teeth
K01.1 Impacted teeth
K05.20 Aggressive periodontitis, unspecified
K05.21 Aggressive periodontitis, localized
K09.0 Developmental odontogenic cysts

L03.90 Cellulitis, unspecified

R69 Illness, unspecified

ORAL & MAXILLOFACIAL SURGERY

Code & Nomenclature	Submission Requirements	Valid Tooth/ Quad/Arch/ Surface
D7251 coronectomy – intentional partial tooth removal	Pre-op X-ray	17, 32

Intentional partial tooth removal is performed when a neurovascular complication is likely if the entire impacted tooth is removed.

1. Benefited under individual consideration and only for documented probable neurovascular complications such as proximity to the inferior alveolar nerve.

2. This procedure code is not to be submitted for incomplete or failed extractions.

CROSS CODES
D7251Coronectomy - intentional partial tooth removal

41899 Unlisted procedure, dentoalveolar structures

K01.1 Impacted teeth
K05.20 Aggressive periodontitis, unspecified
K05.21 Aggressive periodontitis, localized
K09.0 Developmental odontogenic cysts

L03.90 Cellulitis, unspecified

R69 Illness, unspecified

Other Surgical Procedures D7260 - D7291

Code & Nomenclature	Submission Requirements	Valid Tooth/ Quad/Arch/ Surface
D7260 oroantral fistula closure	Operative Report	1 - 16, UL, UR

Excision of fistulous tract between maxillary sinus and oral cavity and closure by advancement flap.

CROSS CODES
D7260 - Oroantral fistula closure

30580 Repair fistula; oromaxillary (combine with 31030 if antrotomy is included)
30600 Repair fistula; oronasal
31000 Lavage by cannulation; maxillary sinus (antrum puncture or natural ostium)
31299 Unlisted procedure, accessory sinuses
42215 Palatoplasty for cleft palate; major revision

v.2019

ORAL & MAXILLOFACIAL SURGERY

Code & Nomenclature	Submission Requirements	Valid Tooth/ Quad/Arch/ Surface
D7261 primary closure of a sinus perforation	Operative Report	1 - 16, UL, UR

Subsequent to surgical removal of tooth, exposure of sinus requiring repair, or immediate closure of oroantral or oralnasal communication in absence of fistulus tract.

1. Procedure is by report. If submitted with D7241 (removal of impacted tooth, completely bony, with unusual complications) D7261 will be disallowed.

CROSS CODES
D7261 Primary closure of a sinus perforation

30580 Repair fistula; oromaxillary (combine with 31030 if antrotomy is included)
30600 Repair fistula; oronasal
31299 Unlisted procedure, accessory sinuses

K04.8 Radicular cyst
K05.20 Aggressive periodontitis, unspecified
K05.21 Aggressive periodontitis, localized
K09.0 Developmental odontogenic cysts

L03.90 Cellulitis, unspecified

R69 Illness, unspecified

Code & Nomenclature	Submission Requirements	Valid Tooth/ Quad/Arch/ Surface
D7270 tooth reimplantation and/ or stabilization of accidentally evulsed or displaced tooth	X-ray, Narrative	A - T, 1 - 32

Includes splinting and/or stabilization.

1. Includes postoperative care for and removal of splint by the same dentist/dental office.

2. Narrative should indicate all teeth involved and describe the method of stabilization.

CROSS CODES
D7270
Tooth reimplantation and/or stabilization of accidentally evulsed or displaced tooth

21440 Closed treatment of mandibular or maxillary alveolar ridge fracture (separate procedure)
21445 Open treatment of mandibular or maxillary alveolar ridge fracture (separate procedure)
41899 Unlisted procedure, dentoalveolar structures

S02.5XXA
Fracture of tooth (traumatic), initial encounter for closed fracture

ORAL & MAXILLOFACIAL SURGERY

Code & Nomenclature	Submission Requirements	Valid Tooth/ Quad/Arch/ Surface
D7280 Exposure of an unerupted tooth	X-ray	A - T, 1 - 32

An incision is made and the tissue is reflected and bone removed as necessary to expose the crown of an impacted tooth not intended to be extracted.

CROSS CODES
D7280
Exposure of an unerupted tooth

1899 Unlisted procedure, dentoalveolar structures

K00.6 Disturbances in tooth eruption
K01.1 Impacted teeth

Code & Nomenclature	Submission Requirements	Valid Tooth/ Quad/Arch/ Surface
D7282 mobilization of erupted or malpositioned tooth to aid eruption	X-ray	A - T, 1 - 32

To move/luxate teeth to eliminate ankylosis; not in conjunction with an extraction.

1. When performed in conjunction with other surgery in this immediate area, the benefit is disallowed.

   CROSS CODES
   D7282
   Mobilization of erupted or malpositioned tooth to aid eruption

   41899 Unlisted procedure, dentoalveolar structures

   K00.6 Disturbances in tooth eruption
   K01.1 Impacted teeth
   K03.5 Ankylosis of teeth

Code & Nomenclature	Submission Requirements	Valid Tooth/ Quad/Arch/ Surface
D7283 Placement of device to facilitate eruption of impacted tooth	X-ray	A - T, 1 - 32

Placement of an orthodontic bracket, band or other device on an unerupted tooth, after its exposure, to aid in its eruption. Report the surgical exposure separately using D7280.

1. Coverage for this procedure is limited to members who have Orthodontic plan benefits.

   CROSS CODES *(Code Changed 2019-01-01}*
   D7283
   Placement of device to facilitate eruption of impacted tooth

   41899 Unlisted Placement of an attachment on an unerupted tooth, after its exposure, to aid in its eruption. Report the surgical exposure separately using D7280.

   K00.6 Disturbances in tooth eruption
   K01.1 Impacted teeth

ORAL & MAXILLOFACIAL SURGERY

Code & Nomenclature	Submission Requirements	Valid Tooth/ Quad/Arch/ Surface
D7285 incisional biopsy of oral tissue-hard (bone, tooth)	Pathology Report	1 - 32 UA, LA, UL, UR, LL, LR

For partial removal of specimen only. This procedure involves biopsy of osseous lesions and is not used for apicoectomy/periradicular surgery. This procedure does not entail an excision.

1. This service is disallowed when performed in conjunction with an apicoectomy (D3410, D3421, D3425 or D3426), or surgical extraction (D7210), by the same dentist/dental office in the same surgical area and on the same date of service.

2. This service is disallowed if not submitted with a pathology report.

CROSS CODES
D7285 - Incisional biopsy of oral tissue-hard (bone, tooth)
For partial removal of specimen only. This procedure involves biopsy of osseous lesions and is not used for apicoectomy/periradicular surgery. This procedure does not entail an excision.

11100 Biopsy of skin, subcutaneous tissue and/or mucous membrane (including simple closure), unless otherwise listed; single lesion
11101 each separate/additional lesion (List separately in addition to code for primary procedure)

20220 Biopsy, bone, trocar, or needle; superficial (eg, ilium, sternum, spinous process, ribs)
20225 Biopsy, bone, trocar, or needle; deep (eg, vertebral body, femur)
20240 Biopsy, bone, open; superficial (eg, sternum, spinous process, rib, patella, olecranon process, calcaneus, tarsal, metatarsal, carpal, metacarpal, phalanx)
20245 Biopsy, bone, open; deep (eg, humeral shaft, ischium, femoral shaft)

40808 Biopsy, vestibule of mouth
41899 Unlisted procedure, dentoalveolar structures
42104 Excision, lesion of palate, uvula; without closure
42106 Excision, lesion of palate, uvula; with simple primary closure
42107 Excision, lesion of palate, uvula; with local flap closure
82397 Chemiluminescent assay

K04.8 Radicular cyst
K05.20 Aggressive periodontitis, unspecified
K05.21 Aggressive periodontitis, localized

v.2019

ORAL & MAXILLOFACIAL SURGERY

Code & Nomenclature	Submission Requirements	Valid Tooth/ Quad/Arch/ Surface
D7286 incisional biopsy of oral tissue-soft	Pathology Report	1 - 32 UA, LA, UL, UR, LL, LR

For partial removal of an architecturally intact specimen only. This procedure is not used at the same time as codes for apicoectomy/periradicular curettage. This procedure does not entail an excision.

1. This service is disallowed when performed in conjunction with an apicoectomy (D3410, D3421, D3425 or D3426), or extractions by the same dentist/dental office in the same surgical area and on the same date of service.

2. This service is disallowed if not submitted with a pathology report.

CROSS CODES
D7286 - Incisional biopsy of oral tissue-soft
For partial removal of an architecturally intact specimen only. This procedure is not used at the same time as codes for apicoectomy/periradicular curettage. This procedure does not entail an excision.

11100 Biopsy of skin, subcutaneous tissue and/or mucous membrane (including simple closure), unless otherwise listed; single lesion
11101 each separate/additional lesion (List separately in addition to code for primary procedure)

20200 Biopsy, muscle; superficial

20205 Biopsy, muscle; deep
20206 Biopsy, muscle, percutaneous needle

38500 Biopsy or excision of lymph node(s); open, superficial
38505 Biopsy or excision of lymph node(s); by needle, superficial (eg, cervical, inguinal, axillary) 38510 Biopsy or excision of lymph node(s); open, deep cervical node(s) 38520 Biopsy or excision of lymph node(s); open, deep cervical node(s) with excision scalene fat pad

40525 Excision of lip; full thickness, reconstruction with local flap (eg, Estlander or fan)
41100 Biopsy of tongue; anterior two-thirds
41105 Biopsy of tongue; posterior one-third
41108 Biopsy of floor of mouth
40814 Excision of lesion of mucosa and submucosa, vestibule of mouth; with complex repair
41100 Biopsy of tongue; anterior two-thirds
41105 Biopsy of tongue; posterior one-third
41108 Biopsy of floor of mouth
42100 Biopsy of palate, uvula

v.2019

ORAL & MAXILLOFACIAL SURGERY

Code & Nomenclature	Submission Requirements	Valid Tooth/ Quad/Arch/ Surface
D7290 surgical repositioning of teeth	X-ray	1 - 32 A - T

Grafting procedure(s) is/are additional.

1. Coverage for this procedure is limited to members who have Orthodontic Plan Benefits.

CROSS CODES
D7290
Surgical repositioning of teeth=41899 Unlisted procedure, dentoalveolar structures
Grafting procedure(s) is/are additional

To find a place to start to diagnosis you need to ask the patient how long they have had this. Were they born that way or did something happen?

Code & Nomenclature	Submission Requirements	Valid Tooth/ Quad/Arch/ Surface
D7291 transseptal fiberotomy/supra crestal fiberotomy, by report	Operative Report	1 - 32 A - T

The supraosseous connective tissue attachment is surgically severed around the involved teeth. Where there are adjacent teeth, the transseptal fiberotomy of a single tooth will involve a minimum of three teeth. Since the incisions are within the gingival sulcus and tissue and the root surface is not instrumented, this procedure heals by the reunion of connective tissue with the root surface on which viable periodontal tissue is present (reattachment).

1. Coverage for this procedure is limited to members who have Orthodontic plan benefits.

2. Upon review of documentation, the appropriate benefit allowance will be applied.

CROSS CODES
D7291
Transseptal fiberotomy/supra crestal fiberotomy, by report

The supraosseous connective tissue attachment is surgically severed around the involved teeth. Where there are adjacent teeth, the transseptal fiberotomy of a single tooth will involve a minimum of three teeth. Since the incisions are within the gingival sulcus and tissue and the root surface is not instrumented, this procedure heals by the reunion of connective tissue with the root surface on which viable periodontal tissue is present (reattachment).

41899 Unlisted procedure, dentoalveolar structures

ORAL & MAXILLOFACIAL SURGERY

Code & Nomenclature	Submission Requirements	Valid Tooth/ Quad/Arch/ Surface

Alveoloplasty – Preparation of Ridge D7310 - D7321

D7310

UR, UL
LR, LL

alveoloplasty in conjunction with extractions – four or more teeth or tooth spaces, per quadrant

The alveoloplasty is distinct (separate procedure) from extractions. Usually in preparation for a prosthesis or other treatments such as radiation therapy and transplant surgery. Alveoloplasty is included in the fee for surgical extractions (D7210-D7250), and is disallowed if performed by the same dentist/dental office in the same surgical area on the same date of service.

1.   Allowed with D7140 (extraction, erupted tooth or exposed root) in the same quadrant, when periodontal disease is present.

CROSS CODES
D7310
Alveoloplasty in conjunction with extractions - four or more teeth or tooth spaces, per quadrant The alveoloplasty is distinct (separate procedure) from extractions. Usually in preparation for a prosthesis or other treatments such as radiation therapy and transplant surgery.

41870 Periodontal mucosal grafting
41874 Alveoloplasty, each quadrant (specify)

D7311

1 - 32

alveoloplasty in conjunction with extractions – one to three teeth or tooth spaces, per quadrant

The alveoloplasty is distinct (separate procedure) from extractions. Usually in preparation for a prosthesis or other treatments such as radiation therapy and transplant surgery.

1.   Alveoloplasty is included in the fee for surgical extractions, and is disallowed if performed by the same dentist/dental office in the same surgical area on the same date of service as surgical extraction(s) (D7210-7250).

2.   Allowed with simple extraction in same quadrant, when periodontal disease is present.

3.   If more than one tooth, indicate additional teeth numbers in narrative.

CROSS CODES
D7311
alveoloplasty in conjunction with extractions – one to three teeth or tooth spaces, per quadrant

41870   Periodontal mucosal grafting
41874   Alveoloplasty, each quadrant (specify)

v.2019

ORAL & MAXILLOFACIAL SURGERY

Code & Nomenclature	Submission Requirements	Valid Tooth/ Quad/Arch/ Surface

D7320

alveoloplasty not in conjunction with extractions – four or more teeth or tooth spaces, per quadrant

UR, UL, LR, LL

No extractions performed in an edentulous area. See D7310 if teeth are being extracted concurrently with the alveoloplasty. Usually in preparation for a prosthesis or other treatments such as radiation therapy and transplant surgery.

CROSS CODES

D7320
Alveoloplasty not in conjunction with extractions four or more teeth or tooth spaces, per quadrant No extractions performed in an edentulous area. See D7310 if teeth are being extracted concurrently with the alveoloplasty. Usually in preparation for a prosthesis or other treatments such as radiation therapy and transplant surgery.

41874 Alveoloplasty, each quadrant (specify)
K08.20 Unspecified atrophy of edentulous alveolar ridge

D7321

alveoloplasty not in conjunction with extractions – one to three teeth or tooth spaces, per quadrant

1 - 32

No extractions performed in an edentulous area. See D7311 if teeth are being extracted concurrently with the alveoloplasty. Usually in preparation for a prosthesis or other treatments such as radiation therapy and transplant surgery.

1. If more than one tooth, indicate additional teeth numbers in narrative.

CROSS CODES

D7321
Alveoloplasty not in conjunction with extractions - one to three teeth or tooth spaces, per quadrant No extractions performed in an edentulous area. See D7311 if teeth are being extracted concurrently with the alveoloplasty. Usually in preparation for a prosthesis or other treatments such as radiation therapy and transplant surgery.=41874 Alveoloplasty, each quadrant (specify)

K08.20 Unspecified atrophy of edentulous alveolar ridge

ORAL & MAXILLOFACIAL SURGERY

Code & Nomenclature	Submission Requirements	Valid Tooth/ Quad/Arch/ Surface

Excision of Soft Tissue Lesions D7410

General Guidelines

1. Pathology Report should include site and size of growth.

D7410 excision of benign lesion up to 1.25 cm	Medical Carrier Statement, Pathology Report	1 - 32, UA, LA, UR, UL LR, LL

1. The benefit for D7410 is subject to the review of the pathology report and may be included in the benefit for another surgery when performed on the same date of service.

2. This service is disallowed if not submitted with a pathology report.

CROSS CODES

D7410
Excision of benign lesion up to 1.25 cm=11441 Excision, other benign lesion including margins, except skin tag (unless listed elsewhere), face, ears, eyelids, nose, lips, mucous membrane; excised diameter 0.6 to 1.0 cm

11442 Excision, other benign lesion including margins, except skin tag (unless listed elsewhere), face, ears, eyelids, nose, lips, mucous membrane; excised diameter 1.1 to 2.0 cm
21015 Radical resection of tumor (eg, sarcoma), soft tissue of face or scalp; less than 2 cm

40500 Vermilionectomy (lip shave), with mucosal advancement
40510 Excision of lip; transverse wedge excision with primary closure
40520 Excision of lip; V-excision with primary direct linear closure
40810 Excision of lesion of mucosa and submucosa, vestibule of mouth; without repair
40812 Excision of lesion of mucosa and submucosa, vestibule of mouth; with simple repair
40814 Excision of lesion of mucosa and submucosa, vestibule of mouth; with complex repair
40816Excision of lesion of mucosa and submucosa, vestibule of mouth; complex, with excision of underlying muscle
40820 Destruction of lesion or scar of vestibule of mouth by physical methods (eg, laser, thermal, cryo, chemical)
41110 Excision of lesion of tongue without closure
41112 Excision of lesion of tongue with closure; anterior two-thirds
41113 Excision of lesion of tongue with closure; posterior one-third
41114 Excision of lesion of tongue with closure; with local tongue flap
41116 Excision, lesion of floor of mouth
41825 Excision of lesion or tumor (except listed above), dentoalveolar structures; without repair
41826 Excision of lesion or tumor (except listed above), dentoalveolar structures; with simple repair
42100 Biopsy of palate, uvula

K05.5 Other periodontal diseases
K09.0 Developmental odontogenic cysts
M27.49 Other cysts of jaw

ORAL & MAXILLOFACIAL SURGERY

Code & Nomenclature	Submission Requirements	Valid Tooth/ Quad/Arch/ Surface

Excision of Soft Tissue Lesions D7411 - D7415

General Guidelines

1. Pathology Report should include site and size of growth.

D7411 excision of benign lesion greater than 1.25 cm	Medical Carrier Statement, Pathology Report	1 - 32, UA, LA, UR, UL LR, LL

1. The benefit for D7411 is subject to the review of the pathology report and may be included in the benefit for another surgery when performed on the same date of service.

2. This service is disallowed if not submitted with a pathology report.

D7413 excision of malignant lesion up to 1.25 cm	Medical Carrier Statement, Pathology Report	1 - 32, UA, LA, UR, UL LR, LL
D7414 excision of malignant lesion greater than 1.25 cm		

1. This service is disallowed if not submitted with a pathology report.

CROSS CODES

D7411
Excision of benign lesion greater than 1.25 cm
D7413
Excision of malignant lesion up to 1.25 cm
D7414
Excision of malignant lesion greater than 1.25 cm

21030 Excision of benign tumor or cyst of maxilla or zygoma by enucleation and curettage
21040 Excision of benign tumor or cyst of mandible, by enucleation and/or curettage
40500 Vermilionectomy (lip shave), with mucosal advancement
40510 Excision of lip; transverse wedge excision with primary closure
40520 Excision of lip; V-excision with primary direct linear closure
40810 Excision of lesion of mucosa and submucosa, vestibule of mouth; without repair
40812 Excision of lesion of mucosa and submucosa, vestibule of mouth; with simple repair
40814 Excision of lesion of mucosa and submucosa, vestibule of mouth; with complex repair
40816 Excision of lesion of mucosa and submucosa, vestibule of mouth; complex, with excision of underlying muscle
40820 Destruction of lesion or scar of vestibule of mouth by physical methods (eg, laser, thermal, cryo, chemical)
41110 Excision of lesion of tongue without closure
41112 Excision of lesion of tongue with closure; anterior two-thirds
41113 Excision of lesion of tongue with closure; posterior one-third
41114 Excision of lesion of tongue with closure; with local tongue flap
41116 Excision, lesion of floor of mouth
41825 Excision of lesion or tumor (except listed above), dentoalveolar structures; without repair
41826 Excision of lesion or tumor (except listed above), dentoalveolar structures; with simple repair
42100 Biopsy of palate, uvula
42104 Excision, lesion of palate, uvula; without closure
42106 Excision, lesion of palate, uvula; with simple primary closure
42107 Excision, lesion of palate, uvula; with local flap closure
K05.5 Other periodontal diseases
K09.0 Developmental odontogenic cysts
M27.49 Other cysts of jaw

ORAL & MAXILLOFACIAL SURGERY

Code & Nomenclature	Submission Requirements	Valid Tooth/ Quad/Arch/ Surface

Excision of Soft Tissue Lesions D7465

General Guidelines

1. Pathology Report should include site and size of growth.

D7465 destruction of lesion(s), by physical or chemical method, by report	Narrative	1 - 32, UA, LA, UR, UL LR, LL

Examples include using cryo, laser or electro surgery.

1. Narrative should describe lesion and method of destruction.

Excision of Intra-Osseous Lesions D7440 - D7441

1. All procedures are subject to coverage under medical.

2. Pathology Report should include site and size of growth.

D7440 excision of malignant tumor – lesion diameter up to 1.25 cm **D7441** excision of malignant tumor — lesion diameter greater than 1.25 cm	Medical Carrier Statement, Pathology Report	1 - 32, UR, UL, LR, LL, UA, LA

1. This service is disallowed if not submitted with a pathology report.

SEE NEXT PAGE FOR ALL CROSS CODES

ORAL & MAXILLOFACIAL SURGERY

Code & Nomenclature	Submission Requirements	Valid Tooth/ Quad/Arch/ Surface

Excision of Soft Tissue Lesions D7465

Excision of Intra-Osseous Lesions D7440 - D7441

CROSS CODES

D7465
Destruction of lesion(s) by physical or chemical method, by report
Examples include using cryo, laser or electro surgery.
D7440
Excision of malignant tumor - lesion diameter up to 1.25 cm
D7441
Excision of malignant tumor - lesion diameter greater than 1.25 cm

17000 Destruction (eg, laser surgery, electrosurgery, cryosurgery, chemosurgery, surgical curettement), premalignant lesions (eg, actinic keratoses); first lesion
17003 Destruction (eg, laser surgery, electrosurgery, cryosurgery, chemosurgery, surgical curettement), premalignant lesions (eg, actinic keratoses); second through 14 lesions, each (List separately in addition to code for first lesion)
17004 Destruction (eg, laser surgery, electrosurgery, cryosurgery, chemosurgery, surgical curettement), premalignant lesions (eg, actinic keratoses), 15 or more lesions
17280 Destruction, malignant lesion (eg, laser surgery, electrosurgery, cryosurgery, chemosurgery, surgical curettement), face, ears, eyelids, nose, lips, mucous membrane; lesion diameter 0.5 cm or less
17281 Destruction, malignant lesion (eg, laser surgery, electrosurgery, cryosurgery, chemosurgery, surgical curettement), face, ears, eyelids, nose, lips, mucous membrane; lesion diameter 0.6 to 1.0 cm
17282 Destruction, malignant lesion (eg, laser surgery, electrosurgery, cryosurgery, chemosurgery, surgical curettement), face, ears, eyelids, nose, lips, mucous membrane; lesion diameter 1.1 to 2.0 cm reconstruction with local flap (eg, Estlander or fan)

40527 Excision of lip; full thickness, reconstruction with cross lip flap (Abbe-Estlander)
40530 Resection of lip, more than one-fourth, without reconstruction
40810 Excision of lesion of mucosa and submucosa, vestibule of mouth; without repair
40812 Excision of lesion of mucosa and submucosa, vestibule of mouth; with simple repair
40814 Excision of lesion of mucosa and submucosa, vestibule of mouth; with complex repair
40816 Excision of lesion of mucosa and submucosa, vestibule of mouth; complex, with excision of underlying muscle
41110 Excision of lesion of tongue without closure
41112 Excision of lesion of tongue with closure; anterior two-thirds
41113 Excision of lesion of tongue with closure; posterior one-third
41114 Excision of lesion of tongue with closure; with local tongue flap
41116 Excision, lesion of floor of mouth
41825 Excision of lesion or tumor (except listed above), dentoalveolar structures; without repair
41826 Excision of lesion or tumor (except listed above), dentoalveolar structures; with simple repair
41827 Excision of lesion or tumor (except listed above), dentoalveolar structures; with complex repair 42104 Excision, lesion of palate, uvula; without closure
42106 Excision, lesion of palate, uvula; with simple primary closure
42107 Excision, lesion of palate, uvula; with local flap closure

K05.5 Other periodontal diseases
K09.0 Developmental odontogenic cysts
M27.49 Other cysts of jaw

v.2019

ORAL & MAXILLOFACIAL SURGERY

Code & Nomenclature	Submission Requirements	Valid Tooth/ Quad/Arch/ Surface
D7450 removal of benign odontogenic cyst or tumor – lesion diameter up to 1.25 cm	Medical Carrier Statement, Pathology Report	1 - 32, UR, UL, LR, LL, UA, LA
D7451 removal of benign odontogenic cyst or tumor – lesion diameter greater than 1.25 cm		

Odontogenic Cyst – Cyst derived from the epithelium of odontogenic tissue (developmental, primordial).

1. The benefit for D7450 / D7451 is subject to the review of the pathology report and may be included in the benefit for another surgery when performed in the same area of the mouth on the same date of service by the same dentist/dental office.

2. This service is disallowed if not submitted with a pathology report.

Code & Nomenclature	Submission Requirements	Valid Tooth/ Quad/Arch/ Surface
D7460 removal of benign nonodontogenic cyst or tumor – lesion diameter up to 1.25 cm	Medical Carrier Statement, Pathology Report	1 - 32, UR, UL, LR, LL, UA, LA
D7461 removal of benign nonodontogenic cyst or tumor – lesion diameter greater than 1.25 cm		

1. This service is disallowed if not submitted with a pathology report.

CROSS CODES

D7450
Removal of benign odontogenic cyst or tumor - lesion diameter up to 1.25 cm
D7451
Removal of benign odontogenic cyst or tumor - lesion diameter greater than 1.25 cm
D7460
Removal of benign nonodontogenic cyst or tumor - lesion diameter up to 1.25 cm
D7461
Removal of benign nonodontogenic cyst or tumor - lesion diameter greater than 1.25 cm

11441 Excision, other benign lesion including margins, except skin tag (unless listed elsewhere), face, ears, eyelids, nose, lips, mucous membrane; excised diameter 0.6 to 1.0 cm
20680 Removal of implant; deep (eg, buried wire, pin, screw, metal band, nail, rod or plate)
21030 Excision of benign tumor or cyst of maxilla or zygoma by enucleation and curettage
21040 Excision of benign tumor or cyst of mandible, by enucleation and/or curettage
21046 Excision of benign tumor or cyst of mandible; requiring intra-oral osteotomy (eg, locally aggressive or destructive lesion[s])
21047 Excision of benign tumor or cyst of mandible; requiring extra-oral osteotomy and partial mandibulectomy (eg, locally aggressive or destructive lesion[s])

41825 Excision of lesion or tumor (except listed above), dentoalveolar structures; without repair 41826 Excision of lesion or tumor (except listed above), dentoalveolar structures; with simple repair 41827 Excision of lesion or tumor (except listed above), dentoalveolar structures; with complex repair K04.8 Radicular cyst

K05.5 Other periodontal diseases
K09.0 Developmental odontogenic cysts
M27.49 Other cysts of jaw

v.2019

ORAL & MAXILLOFACIAL SURGERY

Code & Nomenclature	Submission Requirements	Valid Tooth/ Quad/Arch/ Surface

Excision of Bone Tissue D7471 – D7490

D7471
removal of lateral exostosis (maxilla or mandible)

Operative Report

1 - 32,
UL, UR,
LL, LR,
UA, LA

CROSS CODES
D7471
Removal of lateral exostosis (maxilla or mandible)

21031 Excision of torus mandibularis
21032 Excision of maxillary torus palatinus

41822 Excision of fibrous tuberosities, dentoalveolar structures
41823 Excision of osseous tuberosities, dentoalveolar structures

---

D7472
removal of torus palatinus

Operative Report

UA

CROSS CODES
D7472
Removal of torus palatinus

21031 Excision of torus mandibularis
21032 Excision of maxillary torus palatinus

M27.49 Other cysts of jaw
M27.8 Other specified diseases of jaws

D7473
removal of torus mandibularis

Operative Report

LL, LR

CROSS CODES
D7473
Removal of torus mandibularis

21029 Removal by contouring of benign tumor of facial bone (eg, fibrous dysplasia)
21030 Excision of benign tumor or cyst of maxilla or zygoma by enucleation and curettage
21031 Excision of torus mandibularis
21032 Excision of maxillary torus palatinus

M27.49 Other cysts of jaw
M27.8 Other specified diseases of jaws

D7485
reduction of osseous tuberosity

Operative Report

UL, UR

CROSS CODES
D7485
Reduction of osseous tuberosity

41823 Excision of osseous tuberosities, dentoalveolar structures

M27.49 Other cysts of jaw
M27.8 Other specified diseases of jaws

v.2019

ORAL & MAXILLOFACIAL SURGERY

Code & Nomenclature	Submission Requirements	Valid Tooth/ Quad/Arch/ Surface
D7490 radical resection of maxilla or mandible	Medical Carrier Statement, Operative Report, Pathology Report	UL, UR, LL, LR

Partial resection of maxilla or mandible; removal of lesion and defect with margin of normal appearing bone. Reconstruction and bone grafts should be reported separately.

1. This service is disallowed if not submitted with a pathology report.

   CROSS CODES
   D7490
   Radical resection of maxilla or mandible

   21045 Excision of malignant tumor of mandible; radical resection
   21245 Reconstruction of mandible or maxilla, subperiosteal implant; partial

   M27.49 Other cysts of jaw

Surgical Incision D7510 - D7560

Code & Nomenclature	Submission Requirements	Valid Tooth/ Quad/Arch/ Surface
D7510 incision and drainage of abscess – intraoral soft tissue	Operative Report	A - T, 1 - 32

Involves incision through mucosa, including periodontal origins.

1. The benefit for D7510 is subject to the review of the operative report and may be included in the benefit for another procedure when performed on the same date of service by the same dentist/dentist office.

2. For benefit purposes, the Operative Report must include a clinical diagnosis, site of incision, instrument used and method of drainage.

Code & Nomenclature	Submission Requirements	Valid Tooth/ Quad/Arch/ Surface
D7511 incision and drainage of abscess – intraoral soft tissue – complicated (includes drainage of multiple fascial spaces)	Medical Carrier Statement, Operative Report	A - T 1 - 32

Incision is made intraorally and dissection is extended into adjacent fascial space(s) to provide adequate drainage of abscess/cellulitis.

1. The benefit for D7511 is subject to the review of the operative report and may be included in the benefit for another procedure when performed on the same date of service by the same dentist/dentist office.

CROSS CODES FOR D7510 & D7511 ON NEXT PAGE

ORAL & MAXILLOFACIAL SURGERY

Code & Nomenclature	Submission Requirements	Valid Tooth/ Quad/Arch/ Surface

Surgical Incision D7510 - D7560

D7520 incision and drainage of abscess – extraoral soft tissue	Operative Report	LL, LR, UL,UR, LA, UA

Involves incision through skin.

1. Incision and drainage of abscess - extraoral soft tissue is a benefit only if dental related infection is present.

2. The benefit is denied if not related to a dental infection.

D7521 incision and drainage of abscess – extraoral soft tissue – complicated (includes drainage of multiple fascial spaces)	Medical Carrier Statement, Operative Report	LL, LR UL,UR LA, UA

Incision is made extraorally and dissection is extended into adjacent fascial space(s) to provide adequate drainage of abscess/cellulitis.

1. This procedure is subject to coverage under medical.

2. Incision and drainage of abscess-extraoral soft tissue is a benefit only if dentally-related infection is present.

3. Upon review of documentation, the appropriate benefit allowance will be applied.

CROSS CODES
D7510
Incision and drainage of abscess - intraoral soft tissue - Involves incision through mucosa, including periodontal origins

D7511
incision and drainage of abscess – intraoral soft tissue – complicated (includes drainage of multiple fascial spaces)
Partial resection of maxilla or mandible; removal of lesion and defect with margin of normal appearing bone
Reconstruction and bone grafts should be reported separately

D7520
Incision and drainage of abscess - extraoral soft tissue Involves incision through skin

D7521
Incision and drainage of abscess - extraoral soft tissue - complicated (includes drainage of multiple fascial spaces)
Incision is made extraorally and dissection is extended into adjacent fascial space(s) to provide adequate drainage of abscess/cellulitis

10060 incision and drainage of abscess (eg, carbuncle, suppurative hidradenitis, cutaneous or subcutaneous abscess, cyst, furuncle, or paronychia); simple or single
10160 Puncture aspiration of abscess, hematoma, bulla, or cyst
10180 Incision and drainage, complex, postoperative wound infection

20000 Incision of soft tissue abscess (eg, secondary to osteomyelitis); superficial
20005 Incision and drainage of soft tissue abscess, subfascial (ie, involves the soft tissue below the deep fascia)

40800 Drainage of abscess, cyst, hematoma, vestibule of mouth; simple
40801 Drainage of abscess, cyst, hematoma, vestibule of mouth; complicated
41000 Intraoral incision and drainage of abscess, cyst, or hematoma of tongue or floor of mouth; lingual

ORAL & MAXILLOFACIAL SURGERY

Code & Nomenclature	Submission Requirements	Valid Tooth/ Quad/Arch/ Surface
D7530 removal of foreign body from mucosa, skin, or subcutaneous alveolar tissue	Medical Carrier Statement, Operative Report	A - T, 1 - 32
D7540 removal of reaction producing foreign bodies, musculoskeletal system	Operative Report	A - T, 1 - 32

May include, but is not limited to, removal of splinters, pieces of wire, etc., from muscle and/or bone.

Code & Nomenclature	Submission Requirements	Valid Tooth/ Quad/Arch/ Surface
D7550 partial ostectomy/ sequestrectomy for removal of non-vital bone	Operative Report	A - T, 1 - 32

Removal of loose or sloughed-off dead bone caused by infection or reduced blood supply.

CROSS CODES FOR D7530 & D7540 & D7550
D7530
Removal of foreign body from mucosa, skin, or subcutaneous alveolar tissue

D7540
Removal of reaction producing foreign bodies, musculoskeletal system
May include, but is not limited to, removal of splinters, pieces of wire, etc., from muscle and/or bone

D7550
Partial ostectomy/sequestrectomy for removal of non-vital bone
Removal of loose or sloughed-off dead bone caused by infection or reduced blood supply

10120 Incision and removal of foreign body, subcutaneous tissues; simple
1012 Incision and removal of foreign body, subcutaneous tissues; complicated

20670 Removal of implant; superficial (eg, buried wire, pin or rod) (separate procedure)

40804 Removal of embedded foreign body, vestibule of mouth; simple
40805 Removal of embedded foreign body, vestibule of mouth; complicated
41805 Removal of embedded foreign body from dentoalveolar structures; soft tissues
41806 Removal of embedded foreign body from dentoalveolar structures; bone
41828 Excision of hyperplastic alveolar mucosa, each quadrant (specify)
42809 Removal of foreign body from pharynx

T18.0XXA Foreign body in mouth, initial encounter

Code & Nomenclature	Submission Requirements	Valid Tooth/ Quad/Arch/ Surface
D7560 maxillary sinusotomy for removal of tooth fragment or foreign body	Operative Report	A - T, 1 - 32

CROSS CODES
D7560
Maxillary sinusotomy for removal of tooth fragment or foreign body

31020 Sinusotomy, maxillary (antrotomy); intranasal

31030 Sinusotomy, maxillary (antrotomy); radical (Caldwell-Luc) without removal of antrochoanal polyps
31032 Sinusotomy, maxillary (antrotomy); radical (Caldwell-Luc) with removal of antrochoanal polyps

T18.0XXA Foreign body in mouth, initial encounter

ORAL & MAXILLOFACIAL SURGERY

Code & Nomenclature	Submission Requirements	Valid Tooth/ Quad/Arch/ Surface

Treatment of Closed Fractures - D7610 - D7680

General Guidelines
1. All procedures are subject to coverage under medical.

2. A separate fee for splinting, wiring or banding is disallowed when performed by the same dentist/dental office rendering the primary procedure.

D7610
maxilla – open reduction (teeth immobilized, if present)

Medical Carrier Statement, Operative Report

Teeth may be wired, banded or splinted together to prevent movement. Incision required for interosseous fixation.

D7620
maxilla – closed reduction (teeth immobilized, if present)

Medical Carrier Statement, Operative Report

No incision required to reduce fracture. See D7610 if interosseous fixation is applied.

D7630
mandible – open reduction (teeth immobilized, if present)

Medical Carrier Statement, Operative Report

Teeth may be wired, banded or splinted together to prevent movement. Incision required to reduce fracture.

D7640
mandible – closed reduction (teeth immobilized, if present)

Medical Carrier Statement, Operative Report

No incision required to reduce fracture. See D7630 if interosseous fixation is applied.

CROSS CODES FOR D7610 & D7620 & D7630 & D7640
D7610
Maxilla - open reduction (teeth immobilized, if present)

D7620
Maxilla - closed reduction (teeth immobilized, if present)No incision required to reduce fracture

D7630
Mandible - open reduction (teeth immobilized, if present)

D7640
Mandible - closed reduction (teeth immobilized, if present)

21346 Open treatment of nasomaxillary complex fracture (LeFort II type); with wiring and/or local fixation
21347 Open treatment of nasomaxillary complex fracture (LeFort II type); requiring multiple open approaches
21348 Open treatment of nasomaxillary complex fracture (LeFort II type); with bone grafting (includes obtaining graft)
21422 Open treatment of palatal or maxillary fracture (LeFort I type)
21423 Open treatment of palatal or maxillary fracture (LeFort I type); complicated (comminuted or involving cranial nerve foramina), multiple approaches
21432 Open treatment of craniofacial separation (LeFort III type); with wiring and/or internal fixation
21433 Open treatment of craniofacial separation (LeFort III type); complicated (eg, comminuted or involving cranial nerve foramina), multiple surgical approaches
21435 Open treatment of craniofacial separation (LeFort III type); complicated, utilizing internal and/or external fixation techniques (eg, head cap, halo device, and/or intermaxillary fixation)
21436 Open treatment of craniofacial separation (LeFort III type); complicated, multiple surgical approaches, internal fixation, with bone grafting (includes obtaining graft)
21445 Open treatment of mandibular or maxillary alveolar ridge fracture (separate procedure)
21462 Open treatment of mandibular fracture; with interdental fixation

ORAL & MAXILLOFACIAL SURGERY

Code & Nomenclature	Submission Requirements	Valid Tooth/ Quad/Arch/ Surface

Treatment of Closed Fractures - D7610 - D7680

General Guidelines
1.   All procedures are subject to coverage under medical.

2.   A separate fee for splinting, wiring or banding is disallowed when performed by the same dentist/dental office rendering the primary procedure.

D7650
malar and /or zygomatic arch – open reduction

Medical Carrier Statement,
Operative Report

CROSS CODES
D7650
Malar and/or zygomatic arch - open reduction

21355 Percutaneous treatment of fracture of malar area, including zygomatic arch and malar tripod, with manipulation
21356 Open treatment of depressed zygomatic arch fracture (eg, Gillies approach)
21360 Open treatment of depressed malar fracture, including zygomatic arch and malar tripod
21365 Open treatment of complicated (eg, comminuted or involving cranial nerve foramina) fracture(s) of malar area, including zygomatic arch and malar tripod; with internal fixation and multiple surgical approaches
21366 Open treatment of complicated (eg, comminuted or involving cranial nerve foramina) fracture(s) of malar area, including zygomatic arch and malar tripod; with bone grafting (includes obtaining graft)

40844 Vestibuloplasty; entire arch

D7660
malar and /or zygomatic arch – closed reduction

Medical Carrier Statement,
Operative Report

CROSS CODES
21355   Percutaneous treatment of fracture of malar area, including zygomatic arch and malar tripod, with manipulation
21356   Open treatment of depressed zygomatic arch fracture (eg, Gillies approach)
21360   Open treatment of depressed malar fracture, including zygomatic arch and malar tripod
23155   Excision or curettage of bone cyst or benign tumor of proximal humerus; with autograft (includes obtaining graft)

D7670
alveolus – closed reduction, may include stabilization of teeth

Medical Carrier Statement,
Operative Report,
X-ray

CROSS CODES
21421   Closed treatment of palatal or maxillary fracture (LeFort I type), with interdental wire fixation or fixation of denture or splint
21440   Closed treatment of mandibular or maxillary alveolar ridge fracture (separate procedure)
21445   Open treatment of mandibular or maxillary alveolar ridge fracture (separate procedure)

D7671
alveolus – open reduction, may include stabilization of teeth

Medical Carrier Statement,
Operative Report,
X-ray

CROSS CODES
21422   Open treatment of palatal or maxillary fracture (LeFort I type);
21440   Closed treatment of mandibular or maxillary alveolar ridge fracture (separate procedure)
21445   Open treatment of mandibular or maxillary alveolar ridge fracture (separate procedure)

ORAL & MAXILLOFACIAL SURGERY

Code & Nomenclature	Submission Requirements	Valid Tooth/ Quad/Arch/ Surface

Treatment of Open Fractures –D7710 - D7771

D7710
maxilla – open reduction

Medical Carrier Statement,
Operative Report

Incision required to reduce fracture.

CROSS CODES
21346   Open treatment of nasomaxillary complex fracture (LeFort II type); with wiring and/or local fixation
21347   Open treatment of nasomaxillary complex fracture (LeFort II type); requiring multiple open approaches
21348   Open treatment of nasomaxillary complex fracture (LeFort II type); with bone grafting (includes obtaining graft)
21422   Open treatment of palatal or maxillary fracture (LeFort I type);
21423   Open treatment of palatal or maxillary fracture (LeFort I type); complicated (comminuted or involving cranial nerve foramina), multiple approaches
21432   Open treatment of craniofacial separation (LeFort III type); with wiring and/or internal fixation
21433   Open treatment of craniofacial separation (LeFort III type); complicated (eg, comminuted or involving cranial nerve foramina), multiple surgical approaches
21435   Open treatment of craniofacial separation (LeFort III type); complicated, utilizing internal and/or external fixation techniques (eg, head cap, halo device, and/or intermaxillary fixation)
21436   Open treatment of craniofacial separation (LeFort III type); complicated, multiple surgical approaches, internal fixation, with bone grafting (includes obtaining graft)
21445   Open treatment of mandibular or maxillary alveolar ridge fracture (separate procedure)
21461   Open treatment of mandibular fracture; without interdental fixation
21465   Open treatment of mandibular condylar fracture

D7720
maxilla – closed reduction

Medical Carrier Statement,
Operative Report

CROSS CODES
21345   Closed treatment of nasomaxillary complex fracture (LeFort II type), with interdental wire fixation or fixation of denture or splint
21421   Closed treatment of palatal or maxillary fracture (LeFort I type), with interdental wire fixation or fixation of denture or splint
21431   Closed treatment of craniofacial separation (LeFort III type) using interdental wire fixation of denture or splint
21440   Closed treatment of mandibular or maxillary alveolar ridge fracture (separate procedure)
21450   Closed treatment of mandibular fracture; without manipulation

D7730
mandible – open reduction

Medical Carrier Statement,
Operative Report

Incision required to reduce fracture.

CROSS CODES
21422   Open treatment of palatal or maxillary fracture (LeFort I type);
21445   Open treatment of mandibular or maxillary alveolar ridge fracture (separate procedure)
21452   Percutaneous treatment of mandibular fracture, with external fixation
21454   Open treatment of mandibular fracture with external fixation
21461   Open treatment of mandibular fracture; without interdental fixation
21462   Open treatment of mandibular fracture; with interdental fixation
21465   Open treatment of mandibular condylar fracture
21470   Open treatment of complicated mandibular fracture by multiple surgical approaches including internal fixation, interdental fixation, and/or wiring of dentures or splints

v.2019

ORAL & MAXILLOFACIAL SURGERY

Code & Nomenclature	Submission Requirements	Valid Tooth/ Quad/Arch/ Surface

Treatment of Open Fractures –D7710 - D7771

D7740
mandible – closed reduction

Medical Carrier Statement,
Operative Report

CROSS CODES
21421   Closed treatment of palatal or maxillary fracture (LeFort I type), with interdental wire fixation or fixation of denture or splint
21440   Closed treatment of mandibular or maxillary alveolar ridge fracture (separate procedure)
21450   Closed treatment of mandibular fracture; without manipulation
21451   Closed treatment of mandibular fracture; with manipulation
21452   Percutaneous treatment of mandibular fracture, with external fixation
21453   Closed treatment of mandibular fracture with interdental fixation

D7750
malar and/or zygomatic arch – open reduction

Medical Carrier Statement,
Operative Report

Incision required to reduce fracture.

CROSS CODES
21347   Open treatment of nasomaxillary complex fracture (LeFort II type); requiring multiple open approaches
21348   Open treatment of nasomaxillary complex fracture (LeFort II type); with bone grafting (includes obtaining graft)
21356   Open treatment of depressed zygomatic arch fracture (eg, Gillies approach)
21360   Open treatment of depressed malar fracture, including zygomatic arch and malar tripod
21365   Open treatment of complicated (eg, comminuted or involving cranial nerve foramina) fracture(s) of malar area, including zygomatic arch and malar tripod; with internal fixation and multiple surgical approaches
21366   Open treatment of complicated (eg, comminuted or involving cranial nerve foramina) fracture(s) of malar area, including zygomatic arch and malar tripod; with bone grafting (includes obtaining graft)
21423   Open treatment of palatal or maxillary fracture (LeFort I type); complicated (comminuted or involving cranial nerve foramina), multiple approaches

D7760
malar and/or zygomatic arch – closed reduction

Medical Carrier Statement,
Operative Report

CROSS CODES
21355   Percutaneous treatment of fracture of malar area, including zygomatic arch and malar tripod, with manipulation
21360   Open treatment of depressed malar fracture, including zygomatic arch and malar tripod

ORAL & MAXILLOFACIAL SURGERY

Code & Nomenclature	Submission Requirements	Valid Tooth/ Quad/Arch/ Surface

Treatment of Open Fractures –D7710 - D7771

D7770
alveolus – open reduction stabilization of teeth

Medical Carrier Statement,
Operative Report

Fractured bone(s) are exposed to mouth or outside the face. Incision required to reduce fracture.

CROSS CODES
21422   Open treatment of palatal or maxillary fracture (LeFort I type);
21440   Closed treatment of mandibular or maxillary alveolar ridge fracture (separate procedure)
21445   Open treatment of mandibular or maxillary alveolar ridge fracture (separate procedure)
21453   Closed treatment of mandibular fracture with interdental fixation

D7771
alveolus, closed reduction stabilization of teeth

Medical Carrier Statement,
Operative Report

Fractured bone(s) are exposed to mouth or outside the face.

CROSS CODES
21421   Closed treatment of palatal or maxillary fracture (LeFort I type), with interdental wire fixation or fixation of denture or splint
21440   Closed treatment of mandibular or maxillary alveolar ridge fracture (separate procedure)
21445   Open treatment of mandibular or maxillary alveolar ridge fracture (separate procedure)

ORAL & MAXILLOFACIAL SURGERY

Code & Nomenclature	Submission Requirements	Valid Tooth/ Quad/Arch/ Surface

Reduction of Dislocation and Management of Other Temporomandibular Joint Dysfunctions D7810 - D7830

D7810 open reduction of dislocation	Medical Carrier Statement, Operative Report	

Access to TMJ via surgical opening

1. Coverage is limited to members who have TMJ benefits

D7820 closed reduction of dislocation	Medical Carrier Statement, Operative Report	

Joint manipulated into place; no surgical exposure.

1. Coverage is limited to members who have TMJ benefits.

D7830 manipulation under anesthesia	Medical Carrier Statement, Operative Report	

1. Coverage is limited to members who have TMJ benefits.

CROSS CODES FOR D7810 & D7820 & D7830

D7810
Open reduction of dislocation Access to TMJ via surgical opening

D7820
Closed reduction of dislocation

D7830
Manipulation under anesthesia Usually done under general anesthesia or intravenous sedation.

21480 Closed treatment of temporomandibular dislocation; initial or subsequent
21485 Closed treatment of temporomandibular dislocation; complicated (eg, recurrent requiring intermaxillary fixation or splinting), initial or subsequent
21490 Open treatment of temporomandibular dislocation

M26.60 Temporomandibular joint disorder, unspecified
M26.69 Other specified disorders of temporomandibular joint
M26.89 Other dentofacial anomalies
M77.9 Enthesopathy, unspecified

ORAL & MAXILLOFACIAL SURGERY

Code & Nomenclature	Submission Requirements	Valid Tooth/ Quad/Arch/ Surface

Repair of Traumatic Wounds D7910

Excludes closure of surgical incisions.

D7910
suture of recent small wounds up to 5 cm

Medical Carrier Statement,
Operative Report

Complicated Suturing (Reconstruction Requiring Delicate Handling of Tissues and Wide Undermining for Meticulous Closure)

1. Specify site in operative report.

2. Repair of traumatic wounds is limited to oral structures.

3. Operative report should include diagnosis and treatment.

CROSS CODES
D7910
Suture of recent small wounds up to 5 cm

12011	Simple repair of superficial wounds of face, ears, eyelids, nose, lips and/or mucous membranes; 2.5 cm or less
12013	Simple repair of superficial wounds of face, ears, eyelids, nose, lips and/or mucous membranes; 2.6 cm to 5.0 cm
12020	Treatment of superficial wound dehiscence; simple closure
12021	Treatment of superficial wound dehiscence; with packing
40830	Closure of laceration, vestibule of mouth; 2.5 cm or less
40831	Closure of laceration, vestibule of mouth; over 2.5 cm or complex
41250	Repair of laceration 2.5 cm or less; floor of mouth and/or anterior two-thirds of tongue
41251	Repair of laceration 2.5 cm or less; posterior one-third of tongue
41252	Repair of laceration of tongue, floor of mouth, over 2.6 cm or complex
42180	Repair, laceration of palate; up to 2 cm
42182	Repair, laceration of palate; over 2 cm or complex
42900	Suture pharynx for wound or injury

S09.93XA Unspecified injury of face, initial encounter

ORAL & MAXILLOFACIAL SURGERY

Code & Nomenclature	Submission Requirements	Valid Tooth/ Quad/Arch/ Surface

Other Repair Procedures D7920 - D7999

D7953
bone replacement graft for ridge preservation – per site

1. Bone replacement graft for ridge preservation – per site is denied and the approved amount is collectable from the patient unless it is a group contract specific benefit.

2. Benefit is limited to once in a 24 month period.

CROSS CODES
D7953
Bone replacement graft for ridge preservation - per site
Graft is placed in an extraction or implant removal site at the time of the extraction or removal to preserve ridge integrity (e.g., clinically indicated in preparation for implant reconstruction or where alveolar contour is critical to planned prosthetic reconstruction). Does not include obtaining graft material. Membrane, if used should be reported separately

20900 Bone graft, any donor area; minor or small (eg, dowel or button)
21296 Reduction of masseter muscle and bone (eg, for treatment of benign masseteric hypertrophy); intraoral approach
21299 Unlisted craniofacial and maxillofacial procedure

K08.9 Disorder of teeth and supporting structures, unspecified

---

D7960
frenulectomy – also known as frenectomy or frenotomy – separate procedure not incidental to another procedure

	Narrative	UA, LA, 1 - 32

Removal or release of mucosal and muscle elements of a buccal, labial or lingual that is associated with a pathological condition, or interferes with proper oral development or treatment.

1. Narrative should include diagnosis and clinical indications for the procedure.

2. Frenulectomy is disallowed when performed on the same day in the same surgical area as any periodontal or surgical procedure by the same dentist/dental office.

CROSS CODES
D7960 - Frenulectomy - also known as frenectomy or frenotomy - separate procedure not incidental to another procedure Removal or release of mucosal and muscle elements of a buccal, labial or lingual frenum that is associated with a pathological condition, or interferes with proper oral development or treatment.

40806 Incision of labial frenum (frenotomy)
40819 Excision of frenum, labial or buccal (frenumectomy, frenulectomy, frenectomy)
41010 Incision of lingual frenum (frenotomy)
41115 Excision of lingual frenum (frenectomy)
41520 Frenoplasty (surgical revision of frenum, eg, with Z-plasty)

ORAL & MAXILLOFACIAL SURGERY

Code & Nomenclature	Submission Requirements	Valid Tooth/ Quad/Arch/ Surface

Other Repair Procedures D7920 - D7999

D7963 frenuloplasty	Narrative	UA, LA, 6 -11, 22 - 27

Excision of the frenum with accompanying excision or repositioning of aberrant muscle and z-plasty or other local flap closure.

1. Narrative should include diagnosis and clinical indications for the procedure.

2. Frenuloplasty is disallowed when billed in conjunction with another surgical or periodontal procedure(s) in the same surgical site, by the same dentist/ dental office.

CROSS CODES
D7963
Frenuloplasty Excision of frenum with accompanying excision or repositioning of aberrant muscle and z-plasty or other local flap closure.

41010 Incision of lingual frenum (frenotomy)
41115 Excision of lingual frenum (frenectomy)
41520 Frenoplasty (surgical revision of frenum, eg, with Z-plasty)

K13.70 Unspecified lesions of oral mucosa

M26.30 Unspecified anomaly of tooth position of fully erupted tooth or teeth

---

D7970 excision of hyperplastic tissue – per arch	Narrative	UA, LA

1. The benefit for excision of hyperplastic tissue is disallowed when billed in conjunction with other surgical procedure(s) in the same surgical area by the same dentist/dental office.

2. Limited to edentulous areas.

CROSS CODES
D7970
Excision of hyperplastic tissue - per arch

11440 Excision, other benign lesion including margins, except skin tag (unless listed elsewhere), face, ears, eyelids, nose, lips, mucous membrane; excised diameter 0.5 cm or less
11441 Excision, other benign lesion including margins, except skin tag (unless listed elsewhere), face, ears, eyelids, nose, lips, mucous membrane; excised diameter 0.6 to 1.0 cm
11442 Excision, other benign lesion including margins, except skin tag (unless listed elsewhere), face, ears, eyelids, nose, lips, mucous membrane; excised diameter 1.1 to 2.0 cm
11443 Excision, other benign lesion including margins, except skin tag (unless listed elsewhere), face, ears, eyelids, nose, lips, mucous membrane; excised diameter 2.1 to 3.0 cm
11444 Excision, other benign lesion including margins, except skin tag (unless listed elsewhere), face, ears, eyelids, nose, lips, mucous membrane; excised diameter 3.1 to 4.0 cm
11446 Excision, other benign lesion including margins, except skin tag (unless listed elsewhere), face, ears, eyelids, nose, lips, mucous membrane; excised diameter over 4.0 cm

41828 Excision of hyperplastic alveolar mucosa, each quadrant (specify)

ORAL & MAXILLOFACIAL SURGERY

Code & Nomenclature	Submission Requirements	Valid Tooth/ Quad/Arch/ Surface
D7971 excision of pericoronal gingiva	Narrative	1 - 2, 15 - 16, 17 - 18, 31 - 32

Removal of inflammatory or hypertrophied tissues surrounding partially erupted/impacted teeth.

1. The benefit for excision of pericoronal gingiva is disallowed when billed in conjunction with other surgical procedure(s) in the same surgical area by the same dentist/dental office.

2. This procedure is applicable only to the excision of gingival tissue (operculum) distal to the 2nd or 3rd molars.

CROSS CODES

D7971
Excision of pericoronal gingiva

Removal of inflammatory or hypertrophied tissues surrounding partially erupted/impacted teeth.
11440 Excision, other benign lesion including margins, except skin tag (unless listed elsewhere), face, ears, eyelids, nose, lips, mucous membrane; excised diameter 0.5 cm or less
11441 Excision, other benign lesion including margins, except skin tag (unless listed elsewhere), face, ears, eyelids, nose, lips, mucous membrane; excised diameter 0.6 to 1.0 cm
11442 Excision, other benign lesion including margins, except skin tag (unless listed elsewhere), face, ears, eyelids, nose, lips, mucous membrane; excised diameter 1.1 to 2.0 cm
11443 Excision, other benign lesion including margins, except skin tag (unless listed elsewhere), face, ears, eyelids, nose, lips, mucous membrane; excised diameter 2.1 to 3.0 cm
11444 Excision, other benign lesion including margins, except skin tag (unless listed elsewhere), face, ears, eyelids, nose, lips, mucous membrane; excised diameter 3.1 to 4.0 cm
41820 Gingivectomy, excision gingiva, each quadrant
41821 Operculectomy, excision pericoronal tissues
41872 Gingivoplasty, each quadrant (specify)
K05.20 Aggressive periodontitis, unspecified
K05.30 Chronic periodontitis, unspecified

Code & Nomenclature	Submission Requirements	Valid Tooth/ Quad/Arch/ Surface
D7972 surgical reduction of fibrous tuberosity	Medical Carrier Statement, Operative Report	UA, UR, UL

1. The benefit for surgical reduction of fibrous tuberosity is disallowed when billed in conjunction with other surgical procedure(s) in the same surgical area by the same dentist/dental office.

CROSS CODES

D7972
Surgical reduction of fibrous tuberosity

21029 Removal by contouring of benign tumor of facial bone (eg, fibrous dysplasia)
21030 Excision of benign tumor or cyst of maxilla or zygoma by enucleation and curettage
21031 Excision of torus mandibularis

41822 Excision of fibrous tuberosities, dentoalveolar structures
41828 Excision of hyperplastic alveolar mucosa, each quadrant (specify)

ORAL & MAXILLOFACIAL SURGERY

Code & Nomenclature	Submission Requirements	Valid Tooth/ Quad/Arch/ Surface
D7980 sialolithotomy	Medical Carrier Statement, Operative Report	LA, LL, LR

Surgical procedure by which a stone within a salivary gland or its duct is removed either intraorally or extraorally.

CROSS CODES
D7980
Surgical sialolithotomy

42330 Sialolithotomy; submandibular (submaxillary), sublingual or parotid, uncomplicated, intraoral
42335 Sialolithotomy; submandibular (submaxillary), complicated, intraoral
42340 Sialolithotomy; parotid, extraoral or complicated intraoral
42650 Dilation salivary duct

Code & Nomenclature	Submission Requirements	Valid Tooth/ Quad/Arch/ Surface
D7983 closure of salivary fistula	Medical Carrier Statement, Operative Report	UA, UR, UL, LA, LL, LR

Closure of an opening between a salivary duct and/or gland and the cutaneous surface or an opening into the oral cavity through other than the normal anatomic pathway.

CROSS CODES
D7983
Closure of salivary fistula
Closure of an opening between a salivary duct and/or gland and the cutaneous surface, or an opening into the oral cavity through other than the normal anatomic pathway.

42600 Closure salivary fistula
42650 Dilation salivary duct
42660 Dilation and catheterization of salivary duct, with or without injection

K11.6 Mucocele of salivary gland
K11.9 Disease of salivary gland, unspecified

ORAL & MAXILLOFACIAL SURGERY

Code & Nomenclature	Submission Requirements	Valid Tooth/ Quad/Arch/ Surface
D7999 unspecified oral surgery procedure, by report	Operative Report	

Used for procedure that is not adequately described by a code. Describe procedure.

1. Documentation should include a clinical diagnosis, materials used, tooth number, arch, quadrant, or area of the mouth, chair time, intraoral photographic images when available, X-ray images or additional supporting information.

2. Upon review of documentation, the appropriate benefit allowance will be applied.

CROSS CODES
D7999
unspecified oral surgery procedure, by report

14060   Adjacent tissue transfer or rearrangement, eyelids, nose, ears and/or lips; defect 10 sq cm or less
14061   Adjacent tissue transfer or rearrangement, eyelids, nose, ears and/or lips; defect 10.1 sq cm to 30.0 sq cm
20615   Aspiration and injection for treatment of bone cyst
20926   Tissue grafts, other (eg, paratenon, fat, dermis)
20999   Unlisted procedure, musculoskeletal system, general
21110   Application of interdental fixation device for conditions other than fracture or dislocation, includes removal
21137   Reduction forehead; contouring only
21138   Reduction forehead; contouring and application of prosthetic material or bone graft (includes obtaining autograft)
21139   Reduction forehead; contouring and setback of anterior frontal sinus wall
21155   Reconstruction midface, LeFort III (extracranial), any type, requiring bone grafts (includes obtaining autografts); with LeFort I
21160   Reconstruction midface, LeFort III (extra and intracranial) with forehead advancement (eg, mono bloc), requiring bone grafts (includes obtaining autografts); with LeFort I
21172   Reconstruction superior-lateral orbital rim and lower forehead, advancement or alteration, with or without grafts (includes obtaining autografts)
21175   Reconstruction, bifrontal, superior-lateral orbital rims and lower forehead, advancement or alteration (eg, plagiocephaly, trigonocephaly, brachycephaly), with or without grafts (includes obtaining autografts)
21179   Reconstruction, entire or majority of forehead and/or supraorbital rims; with grafts (allograft or prosthetic material)
21180   Reconstruction, entire or majority of forehead and/or supraorbital rims; with autograft (includes obtaining grafts)
21181   Reconstruction by contouring of benign tumor of cranial bones (eg, fibrous dysplasia), extracranial
21182   Reconstruction of orbital walls, rims, forehead, nasoethmoid complex following intra- and extracranial excision of benign tumor of cranial bone (eg, fibrous dysplasia), with multiple autografts (includes obtaining grafts); total area of bone grafting less than 40 sq cm
21183   Reconstruction of orbital walls, rims, forehead, nasoethmoid complex following intra- and extracranial excision of benign tumor of cranial bone (eg, fibrous dysplasia), with multiple autografts (includes obtaining grafts); total area of bone grafting greater than 40 sq cm but less than 80 sq cm
21184   Reconstruction of orbital walls, rims, forehead, nasoethmoid complex following intra- and extracranial excision of benign tumor of cranial bone (eg, fibrous dysplasia), with multiple autografts (includes obtaining grafts); total area of bone grafting greater than 80 sq cm
21296   Reduction of masseter muscle and bone (eg, for treatment of benign masseteric hypertrophy); intraoral approach
21299   Unlisted craniofacial and maxillofacial procedure
41510   Suture of tongue to lip for micrognathia (Douglas type procedure)
42650   Dilation salivary duct
42660   Dilation and catheterization of salivary duct, with or without injection
42665   Ligation salivary duct, intraoral
42960   Control oropharyngeal hemorrhage, primary or secondary (eg, post-tonsillectomy); simple
42961   Control oropharyngeal hemorrhage, primary or secondary (eg, post-tonsillectomy); complicated, requiring hospitalization
42962   Control oropharyngeal hemorrhage, primary or secondary (eg, post-tonsillectomy); with secondary surgical intervention

K04.8   Radicular cyst

v.2019

Clues from the ADA

The most commonly performed procedure in the OMS practice is extraction of wisdom teeth (third molars). Most tooth extractions are subject to dental benefits but upon request may be reviewed against health insurance policies, and if the criteria is met, the claim may be processed retrospectively and paid under the medical insurance.

Radiology services used to identify embedded or impacted teeth include:
70300 Radiologic examination, teeth, single view
70310 Radiologic examination, teeth, partial examination, less than full mouth
70320 Radiologic examination, teeth, complete, full mouth
70355 Orthopantogram (eg, panoramic x-ray)

Diagnoses may include:
K01.0 Embedded teeth
K01.1 Impacted teeth

One payer says: "...extraction of bony impacted teeth and exposure of impacted teeth are not covered under the medical benefits of the Company's Medicare Advantage plans..."

CDT codes include:
D7280 Surgical access of an unerupted tooth
D7283 Placement of device to facilitate eruption of impacted tooth

Q - What is fibroma and how would removal be reported?
A - A fibroma is a benign tumor composed of fibrous or connective tissue.
Available procedure codes:
D7410 excision of benign lesion up to 1.25cm
D7411 excision of benign lesion greater than 1.25cm

Q - What is a torus/exostosis and how would removal be reported?
A - A torus/exostosis is benign overgrowth of bone forming an elevation or protuberance of bone. They can form in the patient's palate, lingual or lateral aspect of the maxilla or mandible.
Available procedure codes:
D7471 removal of lateral exostosis (maxilla or mandible)
D7472 removal of torus palatinus
D7473 removal of torus madibularis

Q - What is a torus/exostosis and how would removal be reported?
A - A torus/exostosis is benign overgrowth of bone forming an elevation or protuberance of bone. They can form in the patient's palate, lingual or lateral aspect of the maxilla or mandible.
Available procedure codes:
D7471 removal of lateral exostosis (maxilla or mandible)
D7472 removal of torus palatinus
D7473 removal of torus madibularis

Q - How do I code removal of mandibular tori?
A - If the bony elevations are located lingually, code "D7473 removal of torus mandibularis" may be reported by quadrant.

Q - What is a torus/exostosis and how would removal be reported?
A - A torus/exostosis is benign overgrowth of bone forming an elevation or protuberance of bone. They can form in the patient's palate, lingual or lateral aspect of the maxilla or mandible.
Available procedure codes:
D7471 removal of lateral exostosis (maxilla or mandible)
D7472 removal of torus palatinus
D7473 removal of torus madibularis

Q - How do I code the use of collagen wound dressing products that promote hemostatis (blood clotting)?
A - There is no procedure code for collagen wound dressing products. Use of collagen may be a component of a procedure such as "D9930 treatment of complications (post-surgical) - unusual circumstances, by report." In other circumstances, depending on the primary procedure performed, code "D7999 unspecified oral surgery procedure, by report" or "D4999 unspecified periodontal procedure, by report" may be reported.

Q - I removed a portion of the patient's fractured tooth, but not the entire tooth, to provide immediate relief of pain. How should I report this procedure?
A - There is no code that specifically refers to removal of a portion of a fractured tooth to relieve pain. When there is no procedure code whose nomenclature and descriptor reflect the service provided, an "unspecified...procedure, by report" code may be considered (e.g., "D7999 unspecified oral surgery procedure, by report").

Q - A patient needed an extraction, and it turned into a very difficult procedure. The doctor removed most of the tooth, but was unable to remove the entire root and the patient was referred to an oral surgeon immediately. Is there a code for a partial extraction?
A - There are no partial extraction codes available. To report this procedure, use code "D7999 unspecified oral surgery procedure, by report."
D0502 - Other oral pathology procedures, by report
D0999 - Unspecified diagnostic procedure, by report
D1999 - Unspecified preventative procedure, by report
D2999 - Unspecified restorative procedure, by report
D3999 - Unspecified endodontic procedure, by report
D4999 - Unspecified periodontal procedure, by report
D5899 - Unspecified removable prosthodontic procedure, by report
D5999 - Unspecified maxillofacial prosthesis, by report
D6199 - Unspecified implant procedure, but report
D6999 - Unspecified fixed prosthodontic procedure, by report
D7899 - Unspecified TMD therapy; by report
D7999 - Unspecified oral surgery procedure, by report
D8999 - unspecified orthodontic procedure, by report
D9999 - Unspecified adjunctive procedure, by report

v.2019

Links2Success is here to support you in the process of becoming an office that provides sleep apnea services to your community. Get in touch with us for training and assistance.

For more information on cross coding dental billing see Christine's publications:

https://tinyurl.com/ChristineTaxinOnAmazon

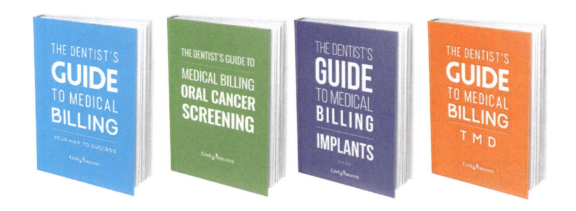

Contact Links2Success for speaking engagements, trainings and other events at

www.links2success.biz

Made in the USA
Middletown, DE
10 June 2021